Department of Veterans Affairs
Health Services Research & Development Service | Evidence-based Synthesis Program

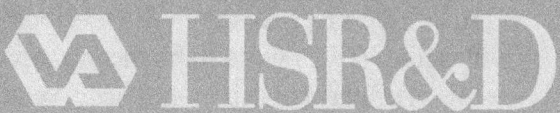

An Overview of Complementary and Alternative Medicine Therapies for Anxiety and Depressive Disorders:

Supplement to Efficacy of Complementary and Alternative Medicine Therapies for Posttraumatic Stress Disorder

I0471951

August 2011

Prepared for:
Department of Veterans Affairs
Veterans Health Administration
Health Services Research & Development Service
Washington, DC 20420

Prepared by:
Evidence-based Synthesis Program (ESP) Center
Durham Veterans Affairs Healthcare System
Durham, NC
John W Williams Jr., M.D., M.H.Sc, Director

Investigators:
John W. Williams Jr., M.D., M.H.Sc.
Jennifer M. Gierisch, Ph.D.
Jennifer McDuffie, Ph.D.
Jennifer L. Strauss, Ph.D.

Research Associate:
  Avishek Nagi, M.S.

Medical Editor:
  Liz Wing, M.A.

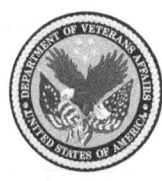

PREFACE

Health Services Research & Development Service's (HSR&D's) Evidence-based Synthesis Program (ESP) was established to provide timely and accurate syntheses of targeted healthcare topics of particular importance to Veterans Affairs (VA) managers and policymakers, as they work to improve the health and healthcare of Veterans. The ESP disseminates these reports throughout VA.

HSR&D provides funding for four ESP Centers and each Center has an active VA affiliation. The ESP Centers generate evidence syntheses on important clinical practice topics, and these reports help:

- develop clinical policies informed by evidence,

- guide the implementation of effective services to improve patient outcomes and to support VA clinical practice guidelines and performance measures, and

- set the direction for future research to address gaps in clinical knowledge.

In 2009, the ESP Coordinating Center was created to expand the capacity of HSR&D Central Office and the four ESP sites by developing and maintaining program processes. In addition, the Center established a Steering Committee comprised of HSR&D field-based investigators, VA Patient Care Services, Office of Quality and Performance, and Veterans Integrated Service Networks (VISN) Clinical Management Officers. The Steering Committee provides program oversight, guides strategic planning, coordinates dissemination activities, and develops collaborations with VA leadership to identify new ESP topics of importance to Veterans and the VA healthcare system.

Comments on this evidence report are welcome and can be sent to Nicole Floyd, ESP Coordinating Center Program Manager, at nicole.floyd@va.gov.

Recommended citation: Williams JW Jr, Gierisch JM, McDuffie J, Strauss JL, Nagi A. An Overview of Complementary and Alternative Medicine Therapies for Anxiety and Depressive Disorders: Supplement to Efficacy of Complementary and Alternative Medicine Therapies for Posttraumatic Stress Disorder. VA-ESP Project #09-010; 2011.

TABLE OF CONTENTS

ABSTRACT

BACKGROUND

VA is committed to expanding the breadth of posttraumatic stress disorder (PTSD)-related services available to Veterans. Since depressive and anxiety disorders share common features with PTSD, this report was commissioned to examine the efficacy of complementary and alternative medicine (CAM) therapies for the treatment of depressive and anxiety disorders as a means to detect treatments that might be applicable to PTSD.

METHODS

The key questions (KQs) were adapted from the parent report, *Efficacy of Complementary and Alternative Medicine Therapies for Posttraumatic Stress Disorder*. We searched MEDLINE® (via PubMed®) and the Cochrane Database of Systematic Reviews for recent English-language systematic reviews (SRs) that examined the literature on mind-body medicine, manipulative and body-based practices, and movement or energy therapies, excluding nutritionals, herbal remedies and other supplements. To be included, SRs had to be published within the past five years and be evaluated as a "fair" or "good" quality. Titles, abstracts, and articles were reviewed in duplicate, and relevant data were abstracted by authors trained in the critical analysis of literature.

KEY FINDINGS

We identified five relevant SRs on mind-body CAM therapies, but none on manipulative and body-based, movement-based, or energy therapies. Most primary studies were small trials that did not provide descriptions of CAM strategies adequate to permit replication. Dose, duration, and frequency of interventions sometimes varied widely. Key findings were:

- For anxiety disorders, there is limited evidence on the effectiveness of meditation (n = 2 studies). Studies reported high rates of dropout, suggesting that adherence to meditation may be problematic in a clinical setting; therefore, it is difficult to draw conclusions about the efficacy of meditation for the treatment of anxiety disorders.

- Relaxation and/or breathing retraining show promise as a CAM therapy for panic disorders. Evidence, however, is limited.

- Acupuncture shows some promise as a CAM therapy for depression, but results were mixed. For major depressive disorder (MDD), acupuncture showed greater effects than sham control on depressive symptoms but did not improve response or remission rates. It did not differ significantly from short-term use of antidepressants. However, for patients with post-stroke depression, acupuncture was more effective than short-term use of antidepressants.

- Mindfulness-based stress reduction has shown positive effects on anxiety and depressive symptoms. However, studies are poor to fair quality.

- No included SRs reported effects on health-related quality of life. Reported results provided limited data on adverse effects or retention rates.

The limitations of the current evidence preclude strong conclusions about specific CAM interventions for the treatment of depressive and anxiety disorders. However, limited evidence supports the use of meditation, relaxation training and/or breathing retraining, and mindfulness-based stress reduction for anxiety, as well as acupuncture for depression. This evidence should be considered together with the direct data on CAM treatments for PTSD when planning further treatment studies.

INTRODUCTION

Posttraumatic stress disorder (PTSD) is an anxiety disorder, and the disorder most frequently associated with combat exposure.[1] An anticipated consequence of our troops' prolonged deployments in Iraq and Afghanistan is an increased incidence of PTSD among returning Veterans. The VA is committed to providing cutting-edge, evidence-based treatment for all Veterans, including those seeking PTSD-related services. Complementary alternative medicine (CAM) interventions are widely requested and used by mental health consumers, including Veterans and active duty personnel. CAM treatments are perceived to be less invasive and to have fewer side effects than traditional therapies and, in some cases, may be more congruent with individual treatment preference.[2-6] VA is committed to expanding the evidence base and breadth of PTSD-related services available to Veterans. To this end, there is growing interest in applications of CAM. This evidence report was commissioned to examine the efficacy of CAM therapies for the treatment of PTSD.

The Durham Evidence-based Synthesis Program (ESP) Center completed a systematic review, *Efficacy of Complementary and Alternative Medicine Therapies for Posttraumatic Stress Disorder*,[7] that included studies of patients with PTSD. In response to a preliminary presentation, stakeholders and attendees requested the review be extended to other disorders related to, or often comorbid with, PTSD. This supplemental report examines CAM therapies for other anxiety diagnoses and depression to better ascertain the potential for CAM therapies in the treatment of PTSD.

BACKGROUND

The National Vietnam Veterans Readjustment Study (NVVRS) found that 98.9 percent of Veterans with PTSD reached criteria for a lifetime comorbid psychiatric diagnosis, suggesting that the co-occurrence of PTSD with other psychiatric diagnoses is a ubiquitous phenomenon.[8] Almost half of men (47.9%) and women (48.5%) in the general population with PTSD meet criteria for major depressive episode.[9] Of the other anxiety disorders, generalized anxiety disorder (GAD) and social phobia are the most likely to co-occur with both PTSD and major depressive disorder (MDD).[10, 11] Further support for the interrelationship of these disorders is the recommendation for *Diagnostic and Statistical Manual of Mental Disorders, 5th edition* to reclassify the "emotional (or internalizing) disorders," to include GAD, unipolar depression, panic disorder, phobic disorders, obsessional states, dysthymic disorders, PTSD and somatoform disorders.[12] In addition, a shared association with abnormalities in the 5-HT transporter gene provides a potential mechanism to explain the clinical observation that antidepressants are effective for a variety of anxiety disorders. Since these disorders share symptoms, possible causative mechanisms, and common psychological and pharmacologic treatments, it is plausible that CAM therapies shown to be effective for depression or an anxiety disorder may be effective for PTSD.

CAM refers to a group of healing techniques not traditionally practiced by Western-trained physicians but traditionally used in the medical systems of other parts of the world. The National Center for Complementary and Alternative Medicine (NCCAM) in the National Institutes of Health (NIH) has proposed a classification system for CAM therapies that includes natural products (e.g., dietary supplements, herbal remedies), mind-body medicine (e.g., meditation, acupuncture), manipulative and body-based practices (e.g., spinal manipulation, massage), whole medical systems (e.g., traditional Chinese or Ayurvedic medicine), and other alternative practices (e.g., light or movement therapy). However, our stakeholders desired to maintain the same restriction on the definition of CAM as was applied to the original report – exclude natural products. Therefore, this supplemental report examines the evidence base for mind-body medicine, manipulative and body-based practices, and movement or energy therapies in the treatment of depressive disorders and anxiety disorders other than PTSD.

METHODS

This review was commissioned by the Department of Veterans Affairs' Evidence-based Synthesis Program. The key questions (KQs) were adapted from the original report, which addressed CAM treatments in patients with PTSD, to address CAM treatments in patients with depressive or anxiety disorders. CAM therapies are classified using categories proposed by the NCCAM, and the KQs reflect this classification:

KQ 1: In adults with depressive or anxiety disorders, are mind-body complementary and alternative medicine therapies (e.g., acupuncture, yoga, meditation) more efficacious than control for PTSD symptoms and quality of life?

KQ 2: In adults with depressive or anxiety disorders, are manipulative and body-based complementary and alternative medicine therapies (e.g., spinal manipulation, massage) more efficacious than control for PTSD symptoms and quality of life?

KQ 3: In adults with depressive or anxiety disorders, are complementary and alternative medicine therapies that are movement-based or involve energy therapies more efficacious than control for PTSD symptoms and quality of life?

ANALYTIC FRAMEWORK

We developed and followed a standard protocol for all steps of this review. Our approach was guided by the analytic framework shown in Figure 1.

Figure 1. Analytic framework

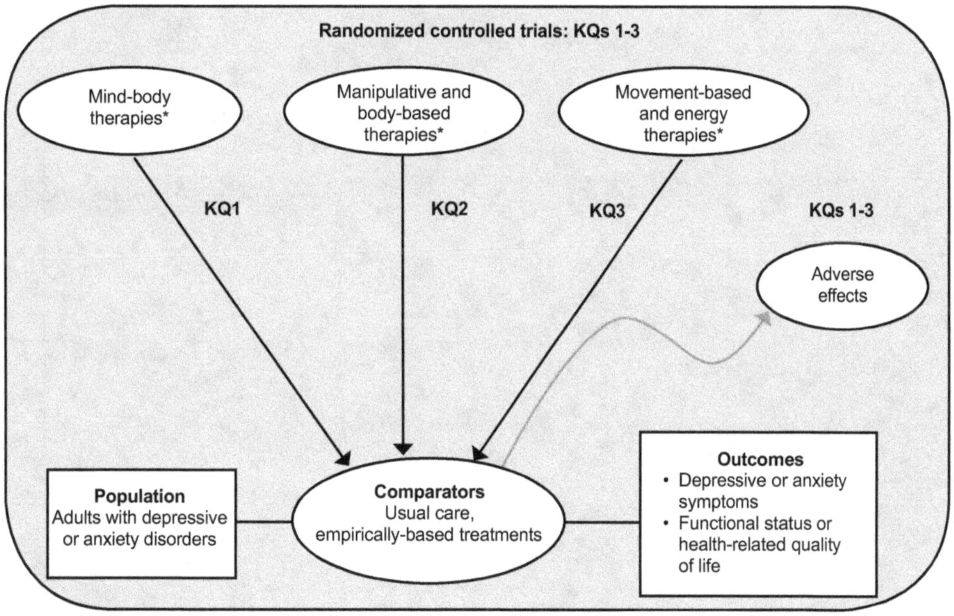

Examples of interventions:

- **Mind-body therapies:** acupuncture, meditation, yoga, deep-breathing exercises, guided imagery, hypnotherapy, progressive relaxation, and tai chi

- **Manipulative and body-based therapies:** spinal manipulation and massage therapy

- **Movement-based therapies:** Feldenkrais method, Alexander technique, Pilates, Rolfing Structural Integration, and Trager Psychophysical Integration

- **Energy therapies:** magnet therapy, light therapy, qi gong, Reiki, and healing touch

SEARCH STRATEGY, STUDY SELECTION AND DATA ABSTRACTION

We searched MEDLINE (via PubMed) and the Cochrane Database of Systematic Reviews for recent English-language SRs that evaluated eligible CAM treatments in patients with a depressive or anxiety disorder excluding PTSD, which was addressed in the main report. Search terms included a validated search filter to identify SRs, terms for eligible CAM treatments, and terms for depressive and anxiety disorders. We used the limit terms Publication Date from 2006/01/01 to 2011/07/01, English, and Humans. Detailed search terms are given in Appendix A. The computerized search was supplemented with a focused review of citations. Using prespecified inclusion/exclusion criteria, two reviewers assessed the list of titles and abstracts. Full-text articles, identified by either reviewer as potentially relevant, were retrieved for further review. Each article retrieved was reviewed by two reviewers using the eligibility criteria in Appendix B; disagreements were resolved by discussion or by a third reviewer. To be included in this report, an SR had to: (1) address one or more eligible CAM treatments in adults with a depressive disorder or anxiety disorder (excluding PTSD), (2) be published within the past 5 years, and (3) be evaluated as a "fair" or "good" quality SR. We used modified Assessment of Multiple Systematic Reviews (AMSTAR) criteria to rate the quality of identified reviews (Appendix C).[13-15] A trained researcher wrote a structured abstract to summarize each review narratively; a second reviewer overread the abstract.

RESULTS

LITERATURE SEARCH

We identified 194 unique SRs from a combined search of MEDLINE (via PubMed with SR filter applied, n = 133) and the Cochrane Database of Systematic Reviews (n = 61). Another potentially relevant review was identified from citations. Of these, 175 were excluded at the title-and-abstract level most often because the population was not adult, the population was not diagnosed with a depressive disorder or anxiety disorder other than PTSD, or the active intervention was not a form of CAM therapy of interest for this report.

An additional 15 studies were excluded following a review of the full text of the 20 articles. Four of these studies were not SRs,[16-19] one was poor quality,[20] four primarily reviewed treatment interventions that were not the CAM therapies of interest[21-24] and six examined populations who were not diagnosed with depressive disorders or an anxiety disorder other than PTSD by valid criteria; e.g., Diagnostic Statistical Manual of Mental Disorders (DSM).[25-30] A table listing these studies and their reasons for exclusion is found in Appendix D. In total, five SRs met eligibility criteria and are summarized by KQ.

KQ 1: In adults with depressive or anxiety disorders, are mind-body complementary and alternative medicine therapies (e.g., acupuncture, yoga, meditation) more efficacious than control for PTSD symptoms and health-related quality of life?

We identified five relevant SRs, two that assessed CAM therapies for depressive disorders,[31, 32] two that assessed CAM therapies for anxiety disorders,[33, 34] and one that assessed CAM therapies for anxiety or depressive disorders.[35] These are summarized below.

Depressive disorders mind-body CAM therapies:

Wang, 2008. Is acupuncture beneficial in depression: A meta-analysis of 8 randomized controlled trials? (Quality rating: Good)

Study summary: The objective of this good-quality report was to synthesize the evidence for the benefit of acupuncture as a treatment for depression. To be eligible for inclusion in this review, studies had to be randomized clinical trials that compared traditional acupuncture as the active intervention with sham acupuncture as the control group in patients with a diagnosis of MDD or depressive neurosis by accepted diagnostic criteria. Acupuncture treatment ranged from 10 to 30 sessions.

Key findings: The authors identified eight small, moderate- to high-quality trials that were included in a meta-analysis (n = 477 patients). Outcome measures were the Hamilton Rating Scale for Depression or the Beck Depression Inventory. A pooled analysis of the depression scores calculated a standardized mean difference (SMD) of -0.65 (95% CI -1.18 to -0.11) indicating greater reduction in depressive symptoms among patients randomized to acupuncture. However, response rates (≥ 50% reduction in symptoms) and remission rates did not differ between active and sham treatments. Six of the eight trials reported response rates for acupuncture compared to sham treatment (RR 1.32; 95% CI 0.83 to 2.10). Remission rates were measured in only four of the eight studies, and no significant difference was found between groups (RR 1.30, 95% CI 0.57 to 2.95).

Considerations: There was a large degree of heterogeneity (I^2 = 67.9 to 84.1%) among the studies: high diversity in the number of sessions; the length of the studies' active treatment phase; the type of randomization; and the type of acupuncture – four had individually chosen sites while the other four used fixed points. The high heterogeneity decreases confidence in the pooled estimate of effect.

Zhang, 2010. The effectiveness and safety of acupuncture therapy in depressive disorders: Systematic review and meta-analysis (Quality rating: Fair)

Study summary: The objective of this fair-quality report was to evaluate the effectiveness of acupuncture as monotherapy and as an additional therapy for depressive conditions. To be eligible for this review, a study needed to be a moderate- to high-quality (Jadad score >3) randomized, controlled trial, and patients had to be diagnosed with MDD by accepted diagnostic criteria or post-stroke depression (PSD) by neuroimaging verification of brain alteration. Acupuncture treatment ranged from 15 to 60 sessions. Control conditions were sham acupuncture (n = 3 MDD; n = 0 PSD), antidepressant medication (n = 15 MDD; n = 12 PSD) or waitlist (n = 1 MDD; n = 3 PSD). Treatment was short term (median = 6 weeks for MDD and 4 weeks for PSD).

Key findings: The review identified 20 trials (n = 1998 patients) on MDD and 15 trials (n = 1680 patients) on PSD. Most trials were conducted in China. In nine trials of MDD (n = 662 patients), there was no significant difference between acupuncture as monotherapy versus antidepressant treatment on change in depressive symptoms (mean difference -0.31, 95% CI -0.94 to 1.56) or response rates (RR = 1.09, 95% CI = 0.92 to 1.30). Other comparisons, acupuncture versus sham acupuncture, waitlist or as adjunctive therapy also did not yield significant differences in response rates. There was some evidence in two trials that acupuncture as an adjunct to antidepressant treatment improved symptom severity (WMD* = 2.38, 95% CI = 0.62 to 4.12) with low heterogeneity (I^2 = 0%), but response rates were not significantly improved. Conversely, for PSD, 11 trials (n = 708) comparing acupuncture as monotherapy versus antidepressant showed a greater response rate for acupuncture (RR† = 1.31, 95% CI = 1.19 to 1.44) with low heterogeneity (I^2 = 0%). Similar effects were obtained for measuring change in symptom severity. Fewer adverse effects were found with acupuncture in 21 of 35 trials reporting this information.

Considerations: There was a large degree of heterogeneity (I^2 = 68-94%) in most comparisons among these trials in the type of acupuncture, the number of acupuncture sessions and the length of treatment (4 to 12 weeks). In 27 of 35 trials, the comparator was antidepressant. Only three of the eight sham controlled trials evaluated by Wang et al.[31] were included in this study. When heterogeneity was controlled by removing outliers, results did not change. Given the degree of heterogeneity, any conclusion about acupuncture as therapy for MDD must be interpreted with caution; however, there is evidence that high-intensity acupuncture may be effective for PSD. Finally, most studies were conducted in China and did not provide detailed information about the study population; therefore, results may not be applicable to U.S. Veterans.

---

* Weighted mean difference
†Relative risk

Hofmann, 2010. The effect of mindfulness-based therapy on anxiety and depression: A meta-analytic review (Quality rating: Fair)

Study Summary: The objective of this fair-quality review was to quantitatively synthesize the evidence on mindfulness-based therapies (MBT) for the treatment of anxiety or depression. To be eligible for this evidence synthesis, studies needed to evaluate mindfulness-based treatment, either mindfulness-based cognitive therapy (MBCT) or mindfulness-based stress reduction (MBSR) in adults age 18 to 65, with a diagnosable psychological or physical/medical disorder and report sufficient data to calculate effect sizes for anxiety and/or depressive outcomes. Comparative and noncomparative studies were included.

Key findings: The review included 39 studies (n = 1,140 patients); primary studies were fair to poor quality (median quality score = 1 on a 0 to 5 point scale, with 5 being highest quality). Of the 39 studies, 16 were controlled studies, and most (n = 11) compared MBT to waitlist or usual care; 15 were conducted in patient samples relevant to this summary (anxiety or depressive disorder). Across all studies, MBT was associated with improved anxiety symptoms (Hedges g 0.63, 95% CI 0.53 to 0.73) and depressive symptoms (Hedges g 0.59, 95% CI 0.51 to 0.66). Extensive sensitivity analysis showed similar effects for those treated with MBCT and MBSR, controlled and uncontrolled studies, and those reporting intent-to-treat analyses.

Considerations: This review evaluated a highly heterogeneous, poor-quality group of studies. Many of the studies used MBCT, a treatment derived from cognitive behavioral therapy and considered to be a mainstream therapy.

Anxiety disorders mind-body CAM therapies:

Krisanaprakornkit, 2006. Meditation therapy for anxiety disorders (Quality rating: Good)

Study summary: The objective of this good-quality report was to synthesize the evidence of meditation therapy for the treatment of anxiety disorders. To be eligible for this evidence review, studies needed to be randomized, controlled trials of concentrative or mindfulness meditation with either an active comparator (i.e., pharmacotherapy, psychological treatments, other meditation methods) or no treatment control.

Key findings: The review identified only two eligible trials,[36, 37] both of moderate quality and conducted in the U.S. Included studies were too varied to pool results. Raskin[36] compared the effectiveness of transcendental meditation, muscle biofeedback, and relaxation training (n = 55). All three conditions reported significant improvement in anxiety symptoms (F = 7.26; df = 1,27; P<0.01), as measured by the Taylor Manifest Anxiety Scale Score. Shannahoff[37] reported on the effectiveness of Kundalini yoga versus mindfulness meditation for participants with obsessive compulsive disorder (n = 21) and found no significant differences on the primary outcome measure (Yale-Brown Obsessive-Compulsive Scale). Two secondary measures, the Perceived Stress Scale and Purpose In Life Scale, showed significant differences favoring Kundalini yoga.

Considerations: Both included studies excluded participants with substance use disorders. Shannahoff[37] also excluded participants who smoked, had spinal/physical issues (e.g., pulmonary disorders, overweight, hypertension, and other cardiovascular issues), or who had another primary psychiatric condition (e.g., MDD, bipolar disorder, schizophrenia). Moreover, dropout rates were high in both studies (44% for Raskin[36] and 33% for Shannahoff[37]).

Sanchez-Meca, 2010. Psychological treatment of panic disorder with or without agoraphobia: A meta-analysis (Quality rating: Fair)

Study summary: The objective of this fair-quality report was to analyze the efficacy of psychological interventions for the treatment of panic disorder with or without agoraphobia. Much of this evidence review focused on non-CAM therapies. Only the CAM-specific results (i.e., relaxation and breathing retraining) are summarized here. To be eligible for this evidence review, studies met the following criteria: recruited participants with panic disorder with no less than five participants, tested psychological treatments only (no adjunctive pharmacotherapy) in experimental arm with a nonactive (e.g., waitlist) or active (e.g., pharmacotherapy, other psychological treatment) comparator, and published between 1980 and 2006 in French or English.

Key findings: Authors identified 42 eligible reports encompassing 65 comparisons. Only three included studies were comparisons of relaxation training and/or breathing retraining (total participants not reported). Relaxation training and breathing retraining improved measures of panic disorder ($d_+ = 0.862$, 95% CI 0.203-1.521) compared to nonactive or active control.

Considerations: This report provided no details on comparator conditions. Also, much of this report is devoted to non-CAM therapies, with only three included studies of CAM-specific therapies. Details on the interventions used were sparse.

KQ 2: In adults with depressive or anxiety disorders, are manipulative and body-based complementary and alternative medicine therapies (e.g., spinal manipulation, massage) more efficacious than control for PTSD symptoms and health-related quality of life?

We found no relevant SRs of good or fair quality.

KQ 3: In adults with depressive or anxiety disorders, are complementary and alternative medicine therapies that are movement-based or involve energy therapies more efficacious than control for PTSD and health-related quality of life?

We found no relevant SRs of good or fair quality.

SUMMARY AND DISCUSSION

We identified five SRs of CAM therapies for depressive and anxiety disorders that were of good or fair quality. All five reviews evaluated mind-body CAM therapies (KQ 1). We found no synthesized evidence of acceptable quality for manipulative and body-based CAM therapies (KQ 2) or CAM movement-based or energy therapies (KQ 3). We summarize the findings below:

- Overall, few recent good- or fair-quality systematic reviews have evaluated CAM therapies of interest for depressive and anxiety disorders.

- For anxiety disorders, there is limited evidence on the effectiveness of meditation (n = 2 studies). Studies reported high rates of dropout, suggesting that adherence to meditation may be problematic in a clinical setting. With so few studies of moderate quality and a small number of participants completing treatments, it is difficult to draw conclusions about the efficacy of meditation for the treatment of anxiety disorders.

- Relaxation and/or breathing retraining show promise as a CAM therapy for panic disorders; however, evidence is limited.

- Acupuncture shows some promise as a CAM therapy for depression; however, results were mixed. For MDD, acupuncture showed greater effects than sham control on depressive symptoms but did not improve response or remission rates. In a fair-quality review, acupuncture did not differ significantly from short-term use of antidepressants. For patients with post-stroke depression, acupuncture was more effective than short-term use of antidepressants.

- Mindfulness-based stress reduction has shown positive effects on anxiety and depressive symptoms; however, studies are poor to fair quality.

- Most SR studies evaluated small trials that did not provide adequate descriptions of CAM strategies to permit replication. Dose, duration, and frequency of interventions sometimes varied widely, which, in turn, influenced estimates of pooled effects.

- No included SRs reported effects on health-related quality of life. Reported results provided limited data on adverse effects or retention rates.

- The limitations of the current synthesized evidence preclude strong conclusions about specific CAM interventions for the treatment of depressive and anxiety disorders. However, limited evidence supports the use of meditation, relaxation training and/or breathing retraining, and mindfulness-based stress reduction for anxiety and acupuncture for depression.

The available evidence on CAM treatments for anxiety or depression has important limitations but identifies a small number of therapies that have at least some evidence of positive effects. This evidence should be considered together with the direct data on CAM treatments for PTSD when planning further treatment studies. Meditation, relaxation and breathing retraining, mindfulness-based stress reduction, and acupuncture showed some limited promise for select populations with anxiety or depressive symptoms. In our review of CAM for PTSD,[7] we found moderate evidence for benefits from acupuncture and low-quality evidence for meditation. Thus, by broadening our review to include closely related conditions, we have identified two additional CAM treatments that should be considered for further evaluation in patients with PTSD.

We did not identify any SRs of good or fair quality that synthesized the evidence for manipulative and body-based CAM therapies or CAM movement-based or energy therapies for depressive and anxiety disorders. Future studies should seek to summarize the available evidence on these CAM modalities; however, a dearth of primary studies may preclude synthesis. As noted in the *Efficacy of Complementary and Alternative Medicine Therapies for Posttraumatic Stress Disorder*[7] report, designing rigorous tests of some CAM modalities may be difficult since sham procedures that are both truly inert and appear sufficiently similar to the active intervention are challenging to devise. Future research may want to test these strategies in small exploratory trials if there is a sufficient theoretical rationale for a beneficial treatment effect.

An Overview of Complementary and Alternative Medicine
Therapies for Anxiety and Depressive Disorders
Evidence-based Synthesis Program

REFERENCES

1.   Friedman MJ. Acknowledging the psychiatric cost of war. *N. Engl. J. Med.* Jul 1 2004;351(1):75-77.

2.   Kessler RC, Davis RB, Foster DF, et al. Long-term trends in the use of complementary and alternative medical therapies in the United States. *Ann. Intern. Med.* Aug 21 2001;135(4):262-268.

3.   Barnes PM, Bloom B, Nahin RL. Complementary and alternative medicine use among adults and children: United States, 2007. *Natl Health Stat Report.* Dec 10 2008(12):1-23.

4.   Unutzer J, Klap R, Sturm R, et al. Mental disorders and the use of alternative medicine: results from a national survey. *A. J. Psychiatry.* Nov 2000;157(11):1851-1857.

5.   Kessler RC, Soukup J, Davis RB, et al. The use of complementary and alternative therapies to treat anxiety and depression in the United States. *A. J. Psychiatry.* Feb 2001;158(2):289-294.

6.   Smith TC, Ryan MA, Smith B, et al. Complementary and alternative medicine use among US Navy and Marine Corps personnel. *BMC Complement Altern Med.* 2007;7:16.

7.   Strauss JL, Coeytaux R, McDuffie J, Nagi A, Williams JWJ. Efficacy of Complementary and Alternative Therapies for Posttraumatic Stress Disorder VA-ESP Project #09-010. 2011.

8.   Badura AS. Theoretical and empirical exploration of the similarities between emotional numbing in posttraumatic stress disorder and alexithymia. *J. Anxiety Disord.* 2003;17(3):349-360.

9.   Kessler RC, Sonnega A, Bromet E, Hughes M, Nelson CB. Posttraumatic stress disorder in the National Comorbidity Survey. *Arch. Gen. Psychiatry.* Dec 1995;52(12):1048-1060.

10.   Brady KT, Clary CM. Affective and anxiety comorbidity in post-traumatic stress disorder treatment trials of sertraline. *Compr. Psychiatry.* Sep-Oct 2003;44(5):360-369.

11.   Dozois DJ, Frewen PA. Specificity of cognitive structure in depression and social phobia: a comparison of interpersonal and achievement content. *J. Affect. Disord.* Feb 2006;90(2-3):101-109.

12.   Goldberg DP, Krueger RF, Andrews G, Hobbs MJ. Emotional disorders: cluster 4 of the proposed meta-structure for DSM-V and ICD-11. *Psychol. Med.* Dec 2009;39(12):2043-2059.

13.   Effectiveness of Continuing Medical Education, Structured Abstract Agency for Healthcare Research and Quality, Rockville, M.D. *http://www.ahrp.gov/clinic/tp/cmetp.htm.* February 2007.

14.   Moher D, Cook DJ, Eastwood S, Olkin I, Rennie D, Stroup DF. Improving the quality of reports of meta-analyses of randomised controlled trials: the QUOROM statement. Quality of Reporting of Meta-analyses. *Lancet.* Nov 27 1999;354(9193):1896-1900.

15.   Shea BJ, Grimshaw JM, Wells GA, et al. Development of AMSTAR: a measurement tool to assess the methodological quality of systematic reviews. *BMC Med Res Methodol.* 2007;7:10.

16.   van der Watt G, Laugharne J, Janca A. Complementary and alternative medicine in the treatment of anxiety and depression. *Curr Opin Psychiatry.* Jan 2008;21(1):37-42.

17.   Halbreich U. Systematic reviews of clinical trials of acupuncture as treatment for depression: how systematic and accurate are they? *CNS Spectr.* Apr 2008;13(4):293-294, 299-300.

18.   Uebelacker LA, Epstein-Lubow G, Gaudiano BA, Tremont G, Battle CL, Miller IW. Hatha yoga for depression: critical review of the evidence for efficacy, plausible mechanisms of action, and directions for future research. *J Psychiatr Pract.* Jan 2010;16(1):22-33.

19.   Teixeira MZ, Guedes CH, Barreto PV, Martins MA. The placebo effect and homeopathy. *Homeopathy.* Apr 2010;99(2):119-129.

20.   Even C, Schroder CM, Friedman S, Rouillon F. Efficacy of light therapy in nonseasonal depression: a systematic review. *J. Affect. Disord.* May 2008;108(1-2):11-23.

21.   Freeman MP, Mischoulon D, Tedeschini E, et al. Complementary and alternative medicine for major depressive disorder: a meta-analysis of patient characteristics, placebo-response rates, and treatment outcomes relative to standard antidepressants. *J. Clin. Psychiatry.* Jun 2010;71(6):682-688.

22.   Li C, He Y, Yu D, Wang J, Omori Ichiro M, Xiao Z. Morita therapy for anxiety disorders. *Cochrane Database of Systematic Reviews.* 2010(7). http://www.mrw.interscience.wiley.com/cochrane/clsysrev/articles/CD008619/frame.html.

23.   Thachil AF, Mohan R, Bhugra D. The evidence base of complementary and alternative therapies in depression. *J. Affect. Disord.* Jan 2007;97(1-3):23-35.

24.   Tsang HW, Chan EP, Cheung WM. Effects of mindful and non-mindful exercises on people with depression: a systematic review. *Br. J. Clin. Psychol.* Sep 2008;47(Pt 3):303-322.

25.   Bohlmeijer E, Prenger R, Taal E, Cuijpers P. The effects of mindfulness-based stress reduction therapy on mental health of adults with a chronic medical disease: a meta-analysis. *J. Psychosom. Res.* Jun 2010;68(6):539-544.

26.   Coelho HF, Boddy K, Ernst E. Massage therapy for the treatment of depression: a systematic review. *Int. J. Clin. Pract.* Feb 2008;62(2):325-333.

27.   Hou WH, Chiang PT, Hsu TY, Chiu SY, Yen YC. Treatment effects of massage therapy in depressed people: a meta-analysis. *J. Clin. Psychiatry.* Jul 2010;71(7):894-901.

28.   Lee MS, Pittler MH, Ernst E. Effects of reiki in clinical practice: a systematic review of randomised clinical trials. *Int. J. Clin. Pract.* Jun 2008;62(6):947-954.

29. Meeks TW, Wetherell JL, Irwin MR, Redwine LS, Jeste DV. Complementary and alternative treatments for late-life depression, anxiety, and sleep disturbance: a review of randomized controlled trials. *J. Clin. Psychiatry.* Oct 2007;68(10):1461-1471.

30. Shih M, Yang YH, Koo M. A meta-analysis of hypnosis in the treatment of depressive symptoms: a brief communication. *Int. J. Clin. Exp. Hypn.* Oct 2009;57(4):431-442.

31. Wang H, Qi H, Wang BS, et al. Is acupuncture beneficial in depression: a meta-analysis of 8 randomized controlled trials? *J. Affect. Disord.* Dec 2008;111(2-3):125-134.

32. Zhang ZJ, Chen HY, Yip KC, Ng R, Wong VT. The effectiveness and safety of acupuncture therapy in depressive disorders: systematic review and meta-analysis. *J. Affect. Disord.* Jul 2010;124(1-2):9-21.

33. Krisanaprakornkit T, Krisanaprakornkit W, Piyavhatkul N, Laopaiboon M. Meditation therapy for anxiety disorders. *Cochrane Database Syst Rev.* 2006(1):CD004998.

34. Sanchez-Meca J, Rosa-Alcazar AI, Marin-Martinez F, Gomez-Conesa A. Psychological treatment of panic disorder with or without agoraphobia: a meta-analysis. *Clin. Psychol. Rev.* Feb 2010;30(1):37-50.

35. Hofmann SG, Sawyer AT, Witt AA, Oh D. The effect of mindfulness-based therapy on anxiety and depression: A meta-analytic review. *J. Consult. Clin. Psychol.* Apr 2010;78(2):169-183.

36. Raskin M, Bali LR, Peeke HV. Muscle biofeedback and transcendental meditation. A controlled evaluation of efficacy in the treatment of chronic anxiety. *Arch. Gen. Psychiatry.* Jan 1980;37(1):93-97.

37. Shannahoff-Khalsa DS, Ray LE, Levine S, Gallen CC, Schwartz BJ, Sidorowich JJ. Randomized controlled trial of yogic meditation techniques for patients with obsessive-compulsive disorder. *CNS Spectr.* Dec 1999;4(12):34-47.

APPENDIX A. SEARCH STRATEGIES

Step	Goal	Terms	Result
1	**Anxiety Terms**	(generalized[tiab] AND anxiety[tiab] AND disorder[tiab]) OR "generalized anxiety disorder" OR "generalised anxiety disorder"[tiab] OR "panic disorder"[tiab] OR "panic disorder"[mesh] OR "phobic disorders"[Mesh] OR agoraphobia[Mesh] OR "obsessive-compulsive disorder"[Mesh] OR "stress disorders, traumatic, acute"[mesh] OR "anxiety disorder NOS"[tiab] OR ("Adjustment Disorder"[tiab] AND anxiety[tiab]) OR "adjustment disorders/therapy"[mesh]	27999
2	**Depression terms**	Depressive disorder[Mesh] OR "subsyndromal depression"[tiab] OR "subthreshold depression"[tiab] OR "minor depression"[tiab]	68923
3	**Interventions**	Acupuncture Therapy[Mesh:noexpl] OR Acupuncture Analgesia[Mesh] OR Acupuncture, Ear[Mesh] OR Electroacupuncture[Mesh] OR Acupuncture[Mesh] OR Acupressure[Mesh] OR Auriculotherapy[Mesh] OR acupuncture[All Fields] OR (acupuncture[All Fields] AND therapy[All Fields]) OR (acupuncture therapy[All Fields]) OR acupressure[All Fields] OR auriculotherapy[All Fields] OR Mind-Body Therapies[Mesh:noexpl] OR Breathing Exercises[Mesh] OR Hypnosis[Mesh] OR Imagery (Psychotherapy)[Mesh] OR Meditation[Mesh] OR Mental Healing[Mesh] OR Relaxation Therapy[Mesh] OR Tai Ji[Mesh] OR Therapeutic Touch[Mesh] OR Yoga[Mesh] OR Mind-Body Relations, Metaphysical[Mesh] OR breath[All Fields] OR breath[All Fields:expl] OR Complementary Therapies[Mesh:noexpl] OR Holistic Health[Mesh] OR Medicine, East Asian Traditional[Mesh] OR Reflexotherapy[Mesh] OR Spiritual Therapies[Mesh] OR acoustics[MeSH] OR acoustics[All Fields] OR acoustic[All Fields] OR aromatherapy [MeSH] OR sensory[All Fields] OR aromatherapy[All Fields] OR art[MeSH] OR art[All Fields] OR colour[All Fields] OR color[MeSH] OR color[All Fields] OR dance[All Fields] OR music[MeSH] OR music[All Fields] OR play and playthings[MeSH] OR (play AND playthings[All Fields]) OR play and playthings[All Fields] OR play[All Fields] OR sensory art therapies[MeSH] OR reflexotherapy[All Fields] OR craniosacral[All Fields] OR magnet[All Fields] OR light[MeSH] OR light[All Fields] OR foldenkrais [Tiab] OR Alexander[Tiab] OR pilates[All Fields] OR trager[All Fields] OR movement therapeutic[All Fields] OR movement therapies[All Fields] OR movement therapy[All Fields] OR healers[All Fields] OR energy[All Fields] OR therapeutic touch[MeSH] OR (therapeutic[All Fields] AND touch[All Fields]) OR therapeutic touch[All Fields] OR reiki[All Fields]) OR ayurvedic[All Fields]	1689320
3	**Study designs**	Cochrane Database Syst Rev [TA] OR search[Title/Abstract] OR meta-analysis[Publication Type] OR MEDLINE[Title/abstract] OR (systematic[Title/Abstract] AND review[Title/Abstract]) OR Systematic[sb]	271733
4	**Combine results and apply limits**	(#1 OR #2) AND #3 AND #4 LIMITS: English and Human and Years 2006-7/1/2011	133

APPENDIX B. ELIGIBILITY CRITERIA

Study characteristic	Inclusion criteria	Exclusion criteria
Study design	Fair- or good-quality systematic review	Non-English language publication Non-peer-reviewed publication
Population	Adults ≥ 19 diagnosed with depressive disorder or anxiety Depressive disorders could include: major depressive disorder, dysthymia, depressive disorder NOS, minor or subthreshold depression Anxiety disorders could include: generalized anxiety disorder, panic disorder, obsessive compulsive disorder, phobic disorders, acute stress disorder, anxiety disorder NOS, adjustment disorder with anxiety or mixed anxiety-depression	Seasonal affective disorder Post-partum depressive disorder Post traumatic stress disorder
Interventions	Any of the following eligible treatments: • Mind-body therapies: acupuncture, meditation, yoga, deep-breathing exercises, guided imagery, hypnotherapy, progressive relaxation, and tai chi • Manipulative and body-based therapies: spinal manipulation and massage therapy • Movement-based therapies: Feldenkrais method, Alexander technique, Pilates, Rolfing Structural Integration, and Trager Psychophysical Integration • Energy therapies: magnet therapy, light therapy, qi gong, Reiki, and healing touch	Interventions used in a continuation or maintenance phase Dietary supplements Standard psychotherapies (e.g., prolonged exposure) and extensions of these therapies (e.g., mindfulness-based cognitive therapy) Relaxation used as a control arm or reported without describing the key components Biofeedback
Comparators	Studies comparing an eligible treatment to a control condition such as usual care (including no treatment), supportive therapy, attention control, sham intervention, or a waitlist Studies comparing an eligible treatment to an empirically based treatment, prolonged exposure, cognitive processing therapy, or antidepressant medication	None
Outcomes	Change in level of depressive or anxiety symptoms (i.e., on self-report and/or clinician-administered measures, including remission rates) or change in quality of life (i.e., functional status and health-related quality of life) Reported at ≥ 6 weeks after treatment initiation	None
Setting	Patients recruited from community or outpatient mental health or general medical settings	None.

Abbreviations: DSM = Diagnostic and Statistical Manual of Mental Disorders, VA = Veterans Affairs

APPENDIX C. STUDY QUALITY ASSESSMENT – SYSTEMATIC REVIEWS*

For reviews, first determine whether it is a systematic review (SR). To be a systematic review, it must include a methods section that describes: (1) a search strategy, and (2) an *a priori* approach to synthesizing the data. For reviews determined to meet the SR criteria, assess methodological quality.

General instructions:

Step 1: Grade each of the criteria listed below as "Yes," "No," "Can't tell" or "Not Applicable". Factors to consider when making an assessment are listed under each criterion. Where appropriate (particularly when assigning a "No," or "Can't tell" score), please provide a brief rationale for your decision (in parentheses).

1. **Is a focused clinical question clearly stated?**

   At a minimum, the question should be developed *a priori* and should clearly identify population and outcomes. The study question does not have to be in PICO (Population, Intervention, Comparisons, Outcomes) format.

2. **Are the search methods used to identify relevant studies clearly described?**

   Search methods described in enough detail to permit replication. (The report must include years and databases used. Key words and/or MeSH terms must be stated and where feasible the search strategy should be provided.)

3. **Was a comprehensive literature search performed?**

   At least two electronic sources should be searched. Electronic searches should be supplemented by consulting: reviews, textbooks, specialized registers, or experts in the field and by reviewing the references in the studies found. (OK to limit to key studies.)

4. **Are the inclusion/exclusion criteria used to screen primary studies clearly described?**

   Inclusion/exclusion criteria described in enough detail to permit replication.

5. **Was there duplicate study selection and data extraction?**

   Did two or more raters make inclusion/exclusion decisions, abstract data, and assess study quality – either independently or with one rater over-reading the first raters result?

   Was an appropriate method used to resolve disagreements (e.g., a consensus procedure)?

6. **Were the characteristics of the included studies provided?**

   In an aggregated form such as a table, data from the original studies should be provided on the participants, interventions and outcomes. The ranges of characteristics in all the studies analyzed (e.g., age, race, sex, relevant socioeconomic data, disease status, duration, severity or other diseases) should be reported.

7. **Was the scientific quality of the included studies assessed and documented?**

   A priori methods of assessment should be provided and criteria used to assess study quality specified in enough detail to permit replication.

8. **Were the methods used to combine the findings of studies appropriate?**

For pooled results, an accepted quantitative method of pooling should be used (i.e., more than simple addition; e.g., random-effects or fixed-effect model). For pooled results, a qualitative and quantitative assessment of homogeneity (Cochran's Q and/or I^2) should be performed.

9. **Was the scientific quality of the included studies used appropriately in formulating conclusions?**

The results of the methodological rigor and scientific quality should be considered in the analysis (e.g. subgroup analyses) and the conclusions of the review, and explicitly stated in formulating recommendations.

10. **Was publication bias assessed?**

Publication bias tested using funnel plots, test statistics (e.g., Egger's regression test), and/or search of trials registry for unpublished studies.

11. **Was the conflict of interest stated?**

Potential sources of support should be clearly acknowledged in both the systematic review and the included studies.

12. **Are the stated conclusions supported by the data presented?**

Step 2: Rate the overall quality of the SR as "Good," "Fair," or "Poor" using the guidance below.

Good = After considering items 1 to 11, item 12 is rated "Yes" with no important limitations. This means that few of the items 1 to 11 are rated "No," and none of the limitations are thought to decrease the validity of the conclusions.

Fair = After considering items 1 to 11, item 12 is rated "Yes," but with at least some important limitations. This means that enough of the items 1 to 11 are rated "No" to introduce some uncertainty about the validity of the conclusions.

Poor = After considering items 1 to 11, item 12 is rated "No." This means that several of items 1 to 11 are rated "No," introducing serious uncertainty about the validity of the conclusions.

* Adapted from:

1.   Effectiveness of Continuing Medical Education, Structured Abstract. February 2007. Agency for Healthcare Research and Quality, Rockville, MD. http://www.ahrq.gov/clinic/tp/cmetp.htm

2.   Moher D, Cook DJ, Eastwood S et al. Improving the quality of reports of meta-analyses of randomized controlled trials: The QUOROM statement. Lancet 1999;354:1896-900.

3.   Shea BJ, Grimshaw JM, Wells GA, Boers M, Andersson N, Hamel C, Porter A, Tugwell P, Moher D, Bouter LM. Development of AMSTAR: a measurement tool to assess the methodological quality of systematic reviews. BMC Medical Research Methodology 2007;7:10.

APPENDIX D: EXCLUDED STUDIES

All studies listed were reviewed in their full-text version and excluded for the reason indicated.

Reference	Design not SR	Intervention not eligible CAM treatment	Population not primary depression or anxiety	Poor quality SR
Bohlmeijer_2010_EN2000			X	
Coelho_2008_EN1926			X	
Even_2008_EN1920				X
Freeman_2010_EN2003		X		
Halbreich_2008_EN1936	X			
Hou_2010_EN1992			X	
Lee_2008_EN1937			X	
Li_2010_EN2066		X		
Meeks_2007_EN1921			X	
Shih_2009_EN1990			X	
Teixeira_2010_EN1998	X			
Thachil_2007_EN1894		X		
Tsang_2008_EN1930		X		
Uebelacker_2010_EN1986	X			
van_der_Watt_2008_EN1932	X			

www.ingramcontent.com/pod-product-compliance
Lightning Source LLC
Chambersburg PA
CBHW081421170526
45166CB00010B/3426